THE POWER OF FAITH

Harness the Power to Create Miracles!

Introduction

Thank you for picking up this book. I'm excited to take you through my story of miracles and the power of faith.

My name is Takahiro Kurogome, born in Tokyo in 1964. I am a ChatGPT seminar instructor.

I had a stroke on November 26, 2023, which left me paralyzed on the right side of my body.

However, with prompt treatment and rehabilitation, I regained the ability to walk and was discharged from the hospital within two weeks. As I continued my home rehabilitation, I gradually became able to write again, and after two months recovered the ability to type on a keyboard. After three months I was completely cured: any lingering symptoms gone.

Do you think that the aftereffects of a stroke cannot be cured?

On the day I was hospitalized, I was shocked to find out from my doctor that once brain cells are destroyed, they cannot be restored. I noticed a change in my body through rehabilitation under the proper guidance of my therapist. I was able to continue rehabilitation happily because I could trust my body. The rehabilitation activated the motor function of my right brain, and the motor function of the right hemisphere of my body recovered.

I have written in this book what I noticed, what kind of rehabilitation I did, how I recovered, how I felt, and the process from the onset of the illness to my recovery.

I used to take my health lightly because of my busy work schedule. I believed I was healthy to begin with, and in my daily life, I only got sick occasionally with headaches and fatigue. I had had an unexpected injury at one point, but it was nothing to be concerned about. I think most people are the same way.

At the annual company physical examination, my blood pressure came out as high the way it did every year, and each time I would have to go see the doctor again, but it was always just a follow-up. I was aware of my lack of exercise. When the doctor asked me about it, I reflexively said that I do a desk job most of the time. As for my weight, people point out that I am too thin for my height, but I have always had this body shape since childhood, and I thought the amount I ate was normal. I have never had any trouble with my weight. I believed I was healthy.

I understand that standard weight is a statistical measure used as a guideline for longevity. However, as a person with a background in science, a lighter body is more energy efficient, a little bit of alcohol makes me feel happy and less stressed, and I don't smoke, so that should have been fine. My Body Mass Index (BMI) is about 18.9, which is within the standard range for weight. The results of my physical examination on June 5, 2023, about eight months before my stroke, also showed no abnormalities, as usual. Nonetheless, I had a stroke.

Upon waking up that Sunday morning, I picked up a pen and attempted to write the date in my notebook, as I always do, while listening to audio SNS Clubhouse. That was when a small anomaly occurred.

"I could not write a word"

I believe my life was given to me so that I talk about this precious experience. I would like to share it with those who think that the aftereffects of a stroke cannot be cured, those who are at risk of having a stroke, and their families, the people with whom they share a home.

To begin, I have compiled a [chronological] list of the major events in my life.

<Chronology>

January 1964: Born in Tokyo. According to my mother, I cried a lot.
December 1969: Parents divorced. Adopted after my mother remarried a self-employed man. Struggled with relationship with adoptive father.
January 1978: In the second year of junior high school, became interested in electricity and studied through correspondence courses. Found a dream for the future.
Mar. 1982 Graduated from Saitama Prefectural Sayama Technical High School←Electrical Department. Admitted to university on recommendation.
August 1983: Built my own computer using electronic components given to me by a college friend.
October 1985: Younger brother (19) died suddenly of subarachnoid hemorrhage while sleeping. I began to struggle with the fear of death.
March 1986: Graduated from the Department of Electrical Engineering, Nippon Institute of Technology.
April 1986: Joined an electronics design and manufacturing company in Tokyo and became an electrical engineer of my dreams.
January 1999: stepfather passes away.

April 2000 Successfully developed an "automatic inspection device" under the direction of the company and received an in-house commendation.

4

August 2002: Resigned from the company due to mental illness caused by overwork caused by rapid increase in development work. Took time off to recuperate.

April 2004: Moved to a printed circuit board design company. In charge of PCB design.

June 2006: Entered the family register with a singer-songwriter. Wedding in Salzburg in August of the same year.

September 2006: Moved to an IT service company, in charge of UPS repair.

September 2007: Moved to an IT trading company in Tokyo. Responsible for technical support of semiconductor products.

Oct. 2007: Birth of first son, bringing the family to a total of three people.

April 2011: Moved to sales. Joined the sales team of a major Japanese manufacturer SI-er company.

March 2014: Father passed away, received a photo and a carpenter's chisel as a memento from stepsister.

June 2020: Read a book that changed my life.

Feb. 2021 Began using Clubhouse, an audio social networking site. Began meeting many people.

August 2021 "44 books I read in the new Corona Disaster: I started to live a richer life through reading + action" published on Kindle

Feb. 2022 Divorce

November 2022: Shocked by the appearance of ChatGPT, started using it

Jan. 2022 Started researching my ancestry. Obtained grandparents' names and dates of birth.

November 11, 2023: Sighted four cars with Zorro license plates in a row for 20 minutes.

November 18, 2023 Attended GifuLabo graduation ceremony and reception

November 23, 2023 Tested positive for influenza A

November 26, 2023 Hospitalized for stroke

December 2023 Discharged from hospital after 2 weeks and continued rehabilitation at home

January 2024 Returned to the hospital. Able to type on a keyboard, began using ChatGPT again.

February 2024: Retired. Completely recovered from the cerebral infarction without any aftereffects.

February 2024 Holds the first ChatGPT seminar

May 2024 Seminar gains 100 participants

June 2024 "The Power of Belief: You too can become a miracle worker! Kindle publication

According to Northwestern Medicine, The probability of fully recovering from a stroke without any aftereffects is 10%. Considering that, I think my recovery can be called a miracle. If my experience can be of help to you, I would be very happy.

Northwestern Medicine:

https://www.nm.org/conditions-and-care-areas/neurosciences/comprehensive-stroke-centers/life-after-stroke

Contents

Introduction.. 1
Contents..7
Chapter 1: The Sudden Stroke.. 10
    The Beginning of Irregularities................................. 10
    EMTs arrive and take me to the hospital................. 14
    Diagnosis and despair..16
Chapter 2: My Family and I... 24
    Childhood Family Environment and Suffering.........25
    Memories of my brother...28
    Death in the Family and Gratitude to the Ancestors... 29
Chapter 3 Work... 32
    The Electrical Engineer of my dreams...................... 32
    Changing Jobs and New Challenges......................... 33
Chapter 4 Encountering CLUBHOUSE..............................36
    The New World of CLUBHOUSE............................... 36
    How to enjoy GIFLabo.. 38
Chapter 5: Days of Rehabilitation...................................... 42
    A Body Heavy Like Lead.. 42
    Rehab Trials and Miracles...45
    The Power of Faith... 48
    Rebirth.. 50
Chapter 6: Learning to Type on the keyboard..................54
    The joy of being able to type on the keyboard......... 54
    Miraculous FACEBOOK LIVE.....................................54
    Walking with Technology Again.................................. 55

The End of a Miracle, a New Beginning 58
Afterword.. 59
External Links...61
Special Acknowledgements.. 62
Author's Profile...67

The Power of Faith

Chapter 1
The Sudden Attack of a Stroke

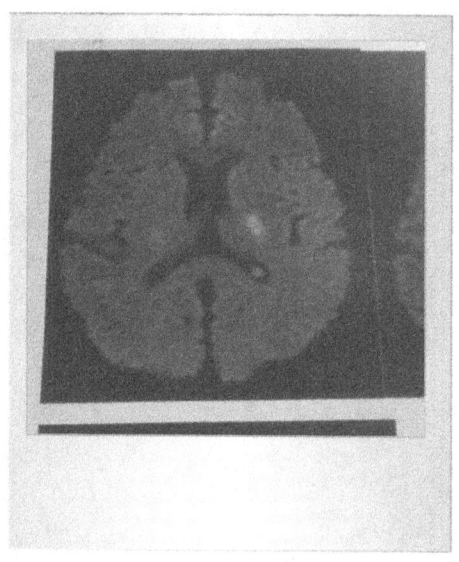

Chapter 1: The Sudden Stroke
The Beginning of Irregularities

It was Sunday, November 26, 2023, around 6:30 in the morning. As is my usual habit, I was listening to the audio social network Clubhouse and trying to write notes in my notebook for the day. I started with the date first. I held the pen in my right hand, placed the nib on the page and tried to write the words, but my right hand would not move properly.

In my head I knew exactly what I was going to write. I knew what day it was, but my hand wouldn't move. The handwriting was so bad that it didn't look like my own. The guest names are indistinguishable. The "2" in the lower left corner of the last letter is not a number at all.

"I can't write…"

For a moment I thought about possible causes, but I had no idea.

Was it because I was sleeping badly and my right hand had been squeezed under my body? I thought for a moment that's what it was, but it was not. There was no pain. I thought I was sleepwalking. Unable to get an answer, I thought something was wrong and felt uneasy. It didn't hurt, but it felt off. It was a strange sensation.

At that moment I had no choice but to stop writing and stand up, my right leg was stiff, my foot got tangled and I almost fell. I quickly grabbed onto the sliding door, but when my body stumbled, the heel of my right foot hit the floor hard enough to bruise and hurt. OUCH! I felt it and knew immediately that I had injured it, but I was surprised to find that I could not move my leg at all, and that was not the point. I didn't care about the sprain.

Why wouldn't it move? Why?

My head was confused. My right leg from the knee down was weak and dangling. I had never experienced my right leg not moving before. The back of my right leg felt pain and I was clearly conscious. What is going on?
I desperately tried to get an idea, but no answer came to me. I stood there and was stunned for a while. At any rate, I went back to my futon, sat down, and settled a bit. I figured that since I could move my left hand and left leg anyway, I could somehow make it to the hospital on my own. Without taking it too seriously, I decided to call a holiday clinic since it was Sunday.

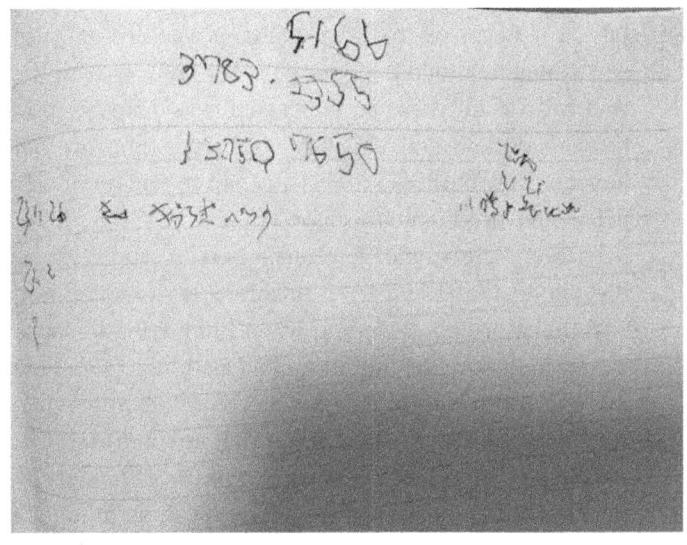

November 26, 2023, my notes. (From left to right: date, Clubhouse room name, guest name

I looked up the phone number for the holiday clinic and called it when it was 9:00 AM. At that time, I was planning to go to the clinic by myself. However, as we talked, I began to feel that walking was not an option and thought about taking a cab. My body was tired. It was a little different from when I was hungry; it was heavier rather than sluggish, and over time my body became less and less mobile. I began to feel anxious, as if I would not be able to move as it was. I was going to need someone's help. I told the person who answered the phone that I had been unable to write since about 6:30 this morning, that even when I did write, the letters would look strange, and that I had a strange tendency to fall over on my right side when I stood up and walked. As I was speaking, feeling somewhat uncomfortable, the person in charge on the other end of the phone seemed to sense the danger and said, "Please call an ambulance and go to the hospital right now!" he said as if shouting. Startled, I hurriedly hung up the phone and immediately dialed 119.

I was asked, "What is the address to which the emergency services will go by dialing 119? I try to speak, but at this point, I am beginning to lose my fluency to the point where I know I am losing it. I wanted him to understand the address somehow, so I tried to repeat it over and over again. I was so desperate to get the message across that I had to restate it three times, but I

13

was becoming increasingly frustrated with myself as my rasping was getting worse. Why can't I speak well? I have never experienced such a frightening thing as this ...... as I become unable to speak during the few minutes I am on the call. My body was slowly breaking down. I felt my life was in danger.

EMTs ARRIVE AND TAKE ME TO THE HOSPITAL

The paramedics instructed me to get ready to be admitted to the hospital and to wait at the door and not to hang up the phone. Thinking quickly, I took only my phone, charger, wallet, and underwear and sat in the doorway and waited.

At this time, I told the ambulance crew that I had tested positive for influenza A a week earlier, on November 23, and that I was still taking my medication as well.

When the ambulance arrived, the crew asked me if I could get in on my own. I said I could, and with my right leg dragging, I walked through the narrow passageway from the front door to the ambulance, which was parked 10 meters away. I was in room 103 at the far end of the first floor, which was inaccessible by stretcher.

In the ambulance, I was asked, "When did your symptoms start?" I answered that it started around 6:30 this morning. The staff explained the reason for the questioning was that it would affect the treatment. The first hospital could not accept the patient, so they stopped and looked for the next hospital. about 5 minutes later, around 9:15, they found the hospital and arrived with sirens at 9:20, about 3 hours after the onset of symptoms.

As we will learn later, there is a time limit from the onset of stroke to the start of treatment for drugs to treat stroke. This is because tPA (tissue plasminogen activator), a drug developed in the United States to dissolve blood clots, increases the frequency of cerebral hemorrhage complications if used more than 4.5 hours after onset. In reality, it takes about one hour after arrival at the hospital for tests and other procedures, so three and a half hours is the actual limit. I was horrified to think that if I had been another 30 minutes later, my chances of recovery would have been even lower.

Upon arrival at the hospital, I was transferred from the stretcher to a bed with a side slide, which was covered around and on top with a transparent plastic sheet for isolation. After blood was immediately drawn and my temperature and blood pressure were taken, I was asked, perhaps as a precaution, "When did the symptoms start?" I was asked. After repeating the same answer, I told him that I had no pain in my head. Shortly after, the attending neurosurgeon quickly appeared and introduced himself. I asked: "Can brain cells regenerate?"; without preamble the neurosurgeon responded:

"Once brain cells are destroyed, they can never be restored."

Diagnosis and despair

For a while, my mind was frozen in shock. Could it be that my body would never heal?

As soon as the conversation was over, as soon as I was lying in bed, an IV drip was started. I was rushed to the MRI room on the first basement floor and moved to the imaging table. The imaging started with a huge noise. I tried not to move.

After the testing was over, the pads holding my head in place were quickly removed and I was swiftly placed on a mobile bed to be taken to a private room on the fifth floor. A short time later, the attending physician reappeared:

"The results of the MRI confirmed that your symptoms are consistent with those of hemiparesis of the right-hand side, so we will be taking a scan every three days to see how you progress."

"I see. .... (I felt discouraged thinking I wouldn't heal anyway).''

I asked my doctor to show me the MRI image a day shortly before I left the hospital.

This is on the 26th. In this image, the body is on its back. The legs are in the front and the head is in the back. The eyes are at the top. This area of about 1 cm, located deep in the center of the left brain, is white (circled in red). This is the area responsible for the right hemisphere's movement, and its white color means that blood flow is low, and it is not functioning. It has not spread to other parts of the brain."

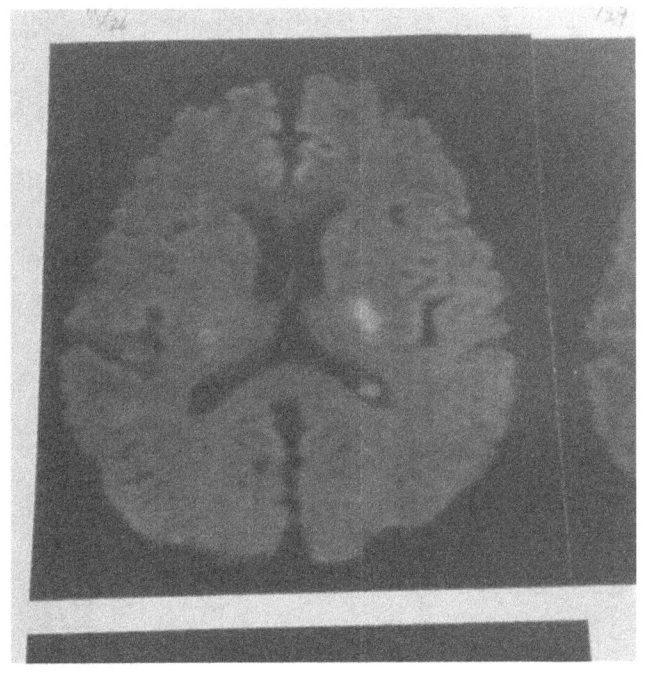

MRI image of the author taken on November 26, shown to him by his doctor

As my doctor left the room, I could hear the faint sound of air conditioning. This room was ventilated. Air entering through the doorway of the room was forced constantly across the bed towards the window at the back of the room.

I looked around to see that it was a rather large private room for one person, with an in-room toilet and shower, and a wheelchair that the nurse had placed beside my bed. The room was chilly, and I looked on my life regretfully as I stared at the IV.

"My body would never heal again."

I wanted to do more. I grieved.

I regretted working for the company.

I should have done more of what I loved.

How did it come to this?

Stress at work?

Anxiety about the coming year?

Too much meat or oil?

Lack of sleep?

Lack of exercise?

I could think of a lot of things, and it was only getting harder. Sighing, I realized with a huff that all my plans had gone out of order, and I knew I had to tell everyone concerned about this situation as soon as possible. I thought I should post it on Facebook, so I took a selfie of myself with an IV drip in my left arm and posted it.

[Author, posting on Facebook November 26, 2023 18:19]

I was hospitalized today for a stroke.

I need rehabilitation.

It will take time to recover, but I will do my best.

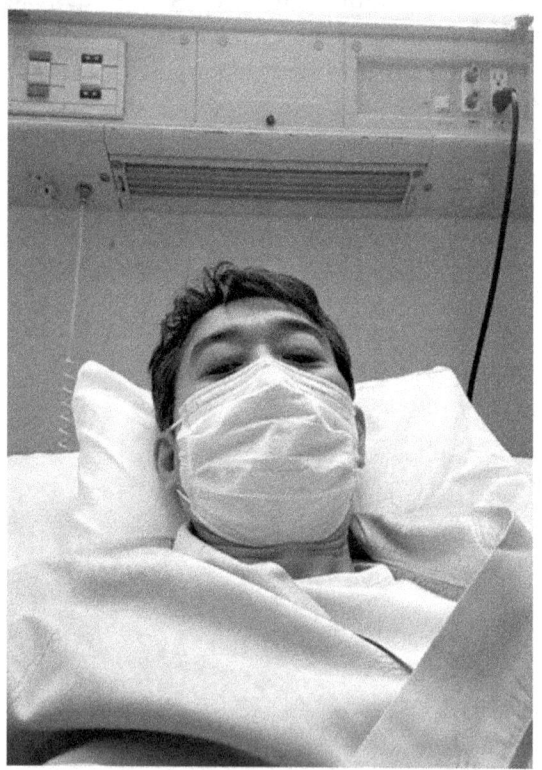

The comments kept coming in from those who saw this short post.

They were all surprised. I am sorry to have surprised you. But I am surprised too that this happened. I posted this as soon as possible to let you know that I can no longer participate in all events. My left arm is in an IV and my right hand, which I believe will never heal, is so heavy that I no longer have the strength to reply.

Akari Taniyama called me immediately with her concern. Akari-san is a fellow Gifulabo listener. We are friends who often work together at events and workshops. I was very happy. She said, "It's all right!" I replied, even though I couldn't understand what she was saying.

On this day, I brought dinner to my mouth as hard as lunch with my left hand and chewed slowly on the left side as if I was treating a cavity. The tongue on the right side did not move well. I accidentally bit my tongue and the pain was relentless. It made me very sad.

After lunch, when I finished brushing my teeth with my left hand, I fell asleep thanks to the gentle strains of Mozart, perhaps because I was tired from the morning.

The next thing that hit me was the fear that I might not even be able to listen to music anymore. The thought that I would never recover made me want to listen to my favorite Mozart on my phone 24 hours a day. As I listened, I kept repeating in my head what my doctor had said. If I never go back to how I was, does that mean the right side of my body will remain immobile?

I spent several days in a private room, but I did not feel that I could move the right side of my body and I thought I would never recover. I couldn't move my right hand properly. I couldn't even take the 5 pills I had to take every morning out of the package, so I had to ask the nurse to take them out for me.

The Power of Faith

Chapter 2
My Family and I

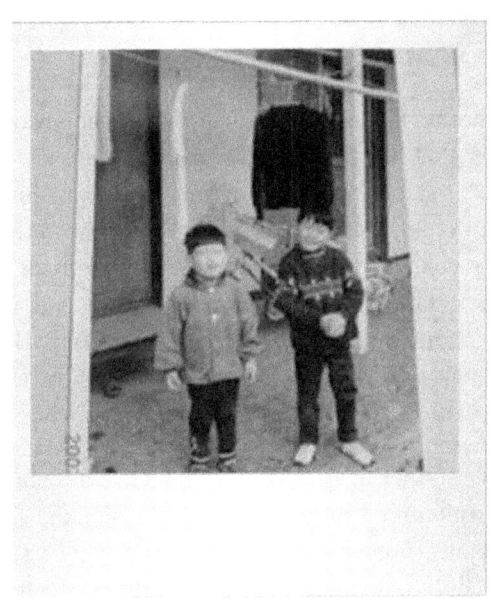

Chapter 2: My Family and I

Childhood Family Environment and Suffering

I was born in Tokyo in January 1964. My father was a carpenter working for the city office in Kodaira, Tokyo. When I was five years old, my parents divorced due to my father's drinking habits and violence. My mother soon remarried, taking me and my three-year-old brother with her.

My mother's second marriage was not happy one, when she felt that her partner was making fun of her for being uneducated, she would snap and yell at him. Since I was a small child, I was afraid of my adoptive father's loud yelling voice, so I was careful not to offend him. My adoptive father's family owned a fruit and vegetable store, and he had many brothers and sisters. He did not get along with his younger siblings and was a loner by nature. He had apparently been a loner at school too.

My stepfather also started his own business in the form of a fruit and vegetable store. He stocked fruits and vegetables, prepared for the opening and closing of the store, but took naps daily, probably because stocking was done as early as 3:00 a.m. He left most of the work to my mother. He would try various ideas on the spur of the moment, but when they didn't work and sales failed, he would change the location and products and start over. At times we ran away from the business at night because we were in such deep debt.

Because of these moves, I attended three elementary schools and three middle schools, six different schools in total. Since I was only in each school for one or two years, I did not fit in, and at one point in middle school I was even bullied. I hardly remember playing with friends, most of my time was spent alone. It was hard at home because I worried about my relationship with my step farther. Friendship with kids my age was also hard, because they were quick to drop me when I moved away. Connecting to people became painful, and it was a heavy load for my mind.

Something happened when I transferred from Saitama Prefecture to a junior high school in Tokyo in my second year of junior high school. I was watching TV and thought to myself, "TVs are not connected by wires, but the pictures move, and the sound comes out. Whoever can design TVs is a genius! I want to be a designer someday. I want to be a designer someday!" I found an ad in a magazine for a correspondence course in electronics, and when I boldly told my mother about it, she paid for it. I can still remember how happy I was.

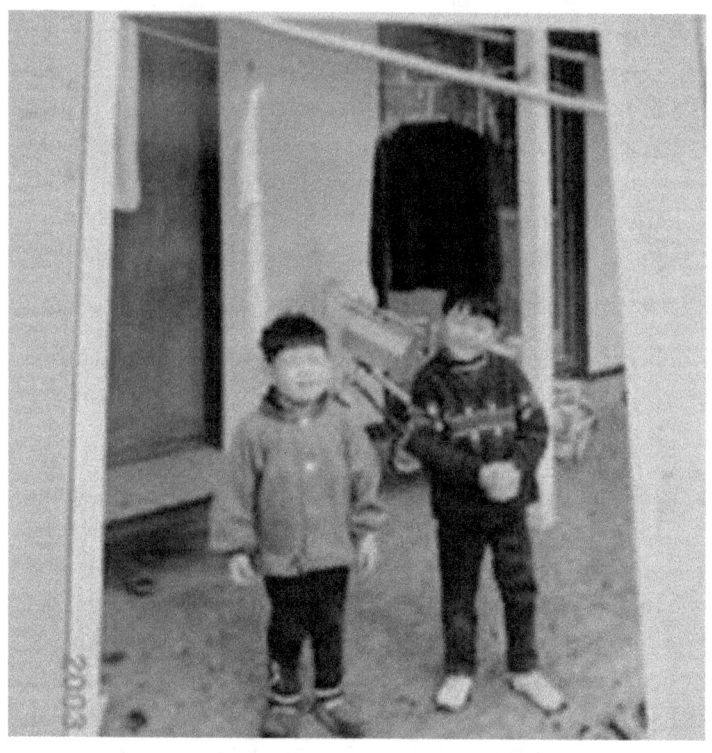

Left: younger brother at around 4 years old,
Right: the author at around 6 years old, photo taken by adoptive father

MEMORIES OF MY BROTHER

My younger brother had a generous personality. I thought he was the type of person who did not talk much, but when I had his birthday analyzed in Yumi Tanabe's "Bebe Fuku-no-Kami Work," I found out that he was a talker. I am not sure if he was not good at studying or if he was unmotivated, but his grades at school were not good. My brother was the type of person who can save money, so I used to target the New Year's money (Otoshidama) he could get. He was the child with the most beautiful handwriting in the family.

My parents worked together and often came home late, so I have strong memories of my younger brother and I always staying at home. I even thought that my parents did not love me at all. I could not tell my mother how uncomfortable I was with my adoptive father. I never told anyone about my parents' divorce or my mother's remarriage.

My younger brother started getting into trouble a lot in middle school. He dropped out of high school as soon as he started, but he attended night school while working part-time.

I have a son, and I feel that he is strangely similar to my brother. He looks like my brother, talks like him, and often finds money on the street. I sometimes wonder if he might be his reincarnation. My son has two friends from elementary school, and even now that he is in high school, the three of us enjoy talking and playing online games together. In short, he is a talkative type.

DEATH IN THE FAMILY AND GRATITUDE TO THE ANCESTORS

My brother did not wake up one Sunday morning.

October 6, 1985. It was Sunday and the family was relaxing. My brother was usually late getting up, but that day, he did not wake up no matter how long it took. When my mother went to his room to wake him up, she screamed. My brother was dead under the covers. He was 19 years old.

The whole family was devastated. The fact that my brother had died of a subarachnoid hemorrhage became a death threat to me, even though I was only 21 years old at the time. I became very afraid of the coming night. I couldn't eat, I was getting thinner and thinner. I was also anxious about university, where I was in the middle of my thesis.

"You don't determine your fate. God does."

This is what I came to understand while I agonized ceaselessly. After realizing this, I felt a little better.

Nothing comes from worrying about death. It is useless to think about it.

In 2014, I received a letter. The sender was from my father's stepdaughter from his second marriage. It was a letter telling me that my father had passed away. I do not remember my father's face at all, nor do I remember having a conversation with him. Through his death, I lost any chance to talk to him again.

Later, she handed me a chisel, a carpenter's tool he had kept as a memento, and a photograph of him, his daughter, and her husband at the park. I felt proud that I had roots in craftsmanship. After visiting the grave of my father, a carpenter craftsman, I began to thank my ancestors before eating my meals.

On November 11, about two weeks before his stroke. I noticed that the license plate numbers of cars passing by were zeroes; if it was just one car, it wouldn't bother me, but within about 20 minutes, I saw four zeros: "55," "00," "99," and "99." I was surprised. I thought it was strange and made a note in my notebook.

The Power of Faith

Chapter 3
Work

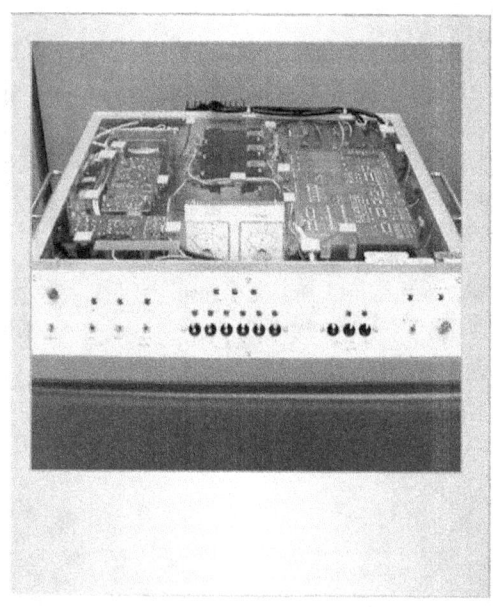

CHAPTER 3 WORK

THE ELECTRICAL ENGINEER OF MY DREAMS

In April 1986, as a new graduate, I entered an electronics design and manufacturing company in Tokyo. I became an electrical engineer, which was my dream job. My first job was designing display boards for radios sold overseas. I was drawing wiring pattern diagrams on special film sheets while learning alongside my seniors. One day, about 14 years after steadily gaining experience as an engineer, I was ordered by the company to develop an automatic inspection system for the production factory line.

Visual checks inevitably lead to mistakes, which is how defective products get missed. I designed the latest computer components, parts by function for product inspection, and circuits for inspection, designed and fabricated circuit boards, assembled the equipment, developed and adjusted control programs, and completed the equipment on my own. My seniors made multiple unsuccessful attempts, but I was the one who managed to complete an automatic inspection device, which had been my long-cherished dream. The device was able to filter out defective products as had been requested. The company was impressed and gave me an award of merit.

After successfully developing the automatic inspection system, the number of development projects for the system increased one after another, and so did my workload. This was because there was no one else who could develop the equipment. After I was transferred from working in an office in Tokyo to working at a factory outside of the prefecture, my commute to work took more than an hour, and I had less time to spend on my work.

At the factory, I was constantly exposed to strong air conditioning, which made me physically ill, and I could not sleep at night because of the cold, so the work piled up.

CHANGING JOBS AND NEW CHALLENGES

After taking a year and a half off, I attempted to change jobs twice, but I struggled to find the right fit, and had to quit soon after starting. On my third attempt, I successfully managed to transfer to an IT trading company. The company was selling semiconductor components and was looking for a technical support person. I was hired because I was familiar with computers and had technical experience. However, sales of these components ended after about a year and a half, and I was once again out of work.

My supervisor told me I have good interpersonal skills and asked me to do an internal help desk for a customer. After two years in this position, I was transferred to a new position and would be a sales representative until retirement. I had no experience in sales, so I joined the sales team of another company and started training from scratch. I had a hard time getting used to it in the beginning, but gradually I adapted. Eventually, I was able to achieve results, such as acquiring new customers at trade show events I attended spontaneously."

With an increase in administrative tasks, I utilized my programming skills to develop a program that extracts necessary data from data files and formats it into the specified file format. This helped streamline administrative work and benefited my sales activities.

Then, just before retirement, as I finished handing over my duties, I suffered a stroke.

The Power of Faith

Chapter 4
Encountering CLUBHOUSE

CHAPTER 4 ENCOUNTERING CLUBHOUSE
THE NEW WORLD OF CLUBHOUSE

Clubhouse, a voice-based social network launched in Japan in late January of 2021 quickly began to gain popularity. I started using it on February 5, having a feeling that it would benefit me somehow. The audio has a warm and friendly feel to it and conveys a lot about people's personalities. I often find myself at real or online events with other listeners, and I feel that strong connection is something that only Clubhouse can provide.

As I continued listening, I noticed two interesting 'rooms': "The 5 a.m. Standard" and "GIFLabo. Both are very informative programs. I have a poor memory so I would write memos in my notebook about the things which I thought would be useful. This is how I started getting up early and jotting notes every morning.

The founder of the "5 a.m. Standard" is Shogo Kotsuka. He is a manager of a listed company and started the program with the intention of training managers at 5 am. Just as his nickname "Iron Man President" suggests, his rules and instructions are strict .

I had made it a habit to get up at 5 a.m., but unfortunately, the "5 a.m. Standard" ended on March 31, 2024. There are no archives (recordings) of the early days, but there are some archives from September 1, 2023 onwards.

I was very happy that Mr. Kotsuka came to visit me while I was in the hospital due to my stroke.

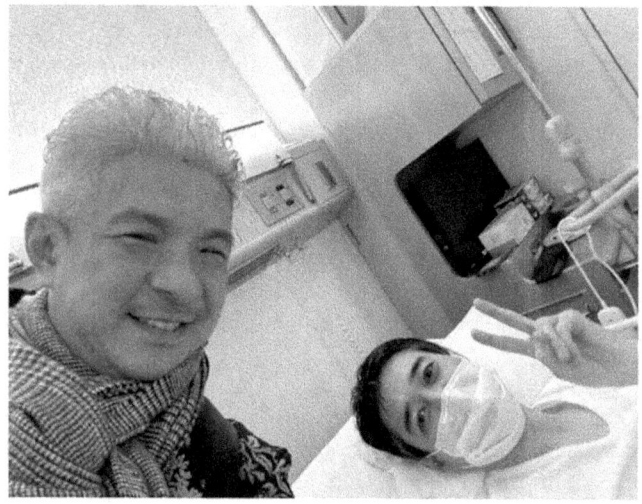

Mr.Kotsuka came to visit me

How to enjoy GIFLabo

The founder of GIFLabO is Mr. Tanakatsu (Katsunari Tanaka). Tanakatsu-san is a communication marketer and the creator of the card game "GIFT". The program starts every morning at around 6:40 am. GIFLabo" stands for Gift Workers Labo.

It was started by Katsunari Tanaka as a way to cheer up those whose sales have plummeted or dropped to zero due to the pandemic. The "room" is fun and laid back, but also thought-provoking, and entertaining, with the moderator actively involved. This unique sense of connection and atmosphere isn't found in other communities or social networks. We invite guests, and moderators, take turns hosting and interviewing them on different days of the week.

One of the nice things about GIFLabo is that it is okay to have moderators dominate the conversation and not give guests an opportunity to speak.

The GIFLabo-Rocket show ended on November 18, 2023, the 1,000th episode of the program. A "graduation ceremony" was held in Tokyo for GIFLabo fans. I attended the ceremony and made a great new memory. When I mentioned that I kept track in my notebook of every episode, Mr. Tanakatsu became curious, which could be taken as his questioning whether there was anything in those discussions worthy of notetaking.

There was. In total I filled 37 notebooks worth of notes. I was happy to be immersed in GIFLabo. It was a wonderful time. I think it's great when everyone gets together and has fun!

It was four days after the graduation ceremony and reception. On November 22, still in the afterglow of the excitement, I became ill with a fever and tested positive for influenza A at the hospital the next day. I was very sad that I could not attend either of the events that I had been looking forward to so much.

(1) "Nov. 22 Animal Fortune-Telling Lab" by Noripi (Ms. Noriko Narita), a GIFLab moderator, 145cm tall, IQ 145, eats 3 pieces of cake a day.

(2)The event will be hosted by Akira (Akira Kashima), a GIFLABO moderator, medium, healer, spiritual YouTube user, and LGBTQ counselor, and Dora-chan (Yoko Morito), another GIFLABO moderator, event and seminar photographer, and Shabu-shabu ambassador (certified manager of Nishi-kawaguchi store). Dora-chan (Yoko Morito), also a Giflab moderator, and a nationwide traveling photographer specializing in events and seminars, and a Shabu-Shabu event on 11/27.

Translated with DeepL.com (free version)

I met so many people through Clubhouse. We connected through Facebook, and so I made many new friends.

When I was hospitalized for my stroke on November 26, I was very happy to receive messages and comments from many people. Their words of sympathy encouraged me and helped me to recover. I would like to take this opportunity to say, 'thank you'.

The Power of Faith

Chapter 5
Days of Rehabilitation

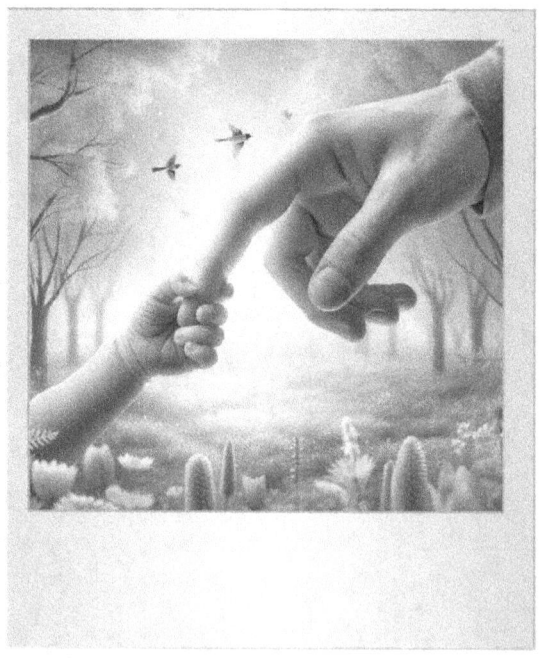

Chapter 5: Days of Rehabilitation
A Body Heavy Like Lead

In this chapter, I describe how rehabilitation helped me overcome the physical and mental barriers I faced. I was able to continue the painful rehabilitation process because I had faith in my body. I will tell you what I realized, what kind of rehabilitation I did, how I recovered, how I felt, and how I went from my situation at the time of admission to my recovery.

I was moved from a private room to a shared room on November 30, one week after I tested positive for influenza A. Rehabilitation started according to the "Rehabilitation Plan" that the physical therapist prepared in advance, based on my condition. The first goal was to recover basic physical functions. The ultimate goal was to regain mobility on the right side of my body. The physical therapist taught me how to move my arms and legs in simple ways.

Each movement is a challenge for the immobile limb at first. Even the slightest of movements is painful. As I lie on the bed, the physical therapist holds my leg and slowly bends then stretches it. I endure the pain with patience, partly out of fear that otherwise I will never be able to move the right side of my body again.

The next day, during the session we go back and forth down the hallway leading to the shared room. The physical therapist accompanies me. I walk carefully and slowly, with my feet not lifting much. I move in a shuffling manner, checking my footing as I walk slowly. I also try moving my right arm, but it feels incredibly heavy, and I quickly become tired. I think, 'Is my arm really this heavy?' It feels like gravity is exerting a strong force on just my right arm.

Now I sit on a bench and lift my right leg. The gravity is so strong that I soon get tired. You realize why astronauts cannot stand up immediately after their return to earth because their muscles are not strong enough to withstand the earth's gravity. I take breaks and move a little at a time, but it is hard, and I want to stop doing it right now. I look around and see other patients in the rehabilitation room silently repeating the same movements as me.

They are lifting their legs, lifting their arms, holding dumbbells and moving their wrists, doing their own routines. No one seems to be enjoying it, since there is not much to say. Strength training in a state of elevated gravity is harder than you might imagine. It feels as if a weight is wrapped around my right arm and leg.

After the morning's entirely unenjoyable workout is over, I quickly finish my eagerly anticipated lunch. Then comes "work" in the afternoon. The occupational therapist in charge comes to the shared room on the 4 floor to get us. We take the elevator down to the second floor together and walk down a long hallway to the workroom in the adjacent rehabilitation ward.

First, we sit in our chairs. The occupational therapist explains the work we are going to do and shows us a model. We are to pinch the edge of the clay with our fingers and pull to stretch it out, making sure we're gripping as strongly as possible.

It seems to be a hard type of clay that is hard to pinch. Pinching and stretching it a little is the most I can do. Next, I pick up the scattered soybeans with chopsticks and transfer them to a bowl. After that, I copy the large letters written in the newspaper onto blank paper. I have never before been praised for my handwriting.

In the evening, it's time for "language." I focus on articulation (pronunciation), starting from a state of slurring the ra-line (of the Japanese syllabary). I practice forming my mouth into shapes like "a," "n," "u," and "i," puffing out my cheeks, moving my tongue in and out of my mouth, rotating it, and repeating short phrases and tongue twisters. It's a practice that can be fun, even if I'm not able to do it perfectly.

The right half of my face is not moving well, making my facial expressions unnatural. My right eyebrow is down, the right eyelid does not close properly, and the right corner of my mouth droops. There is ice in the container brought by the speech therapist. The container looks like a shaker: its tip, round and pointy. Just as I was wondering what it could be used for, when the speech therapist began using it to apply pressure to my face, as though she was writing on it. It was an interesting sensation.

I looked forward to every speech rehab session because I could sit down, not have to move much, and also chat easily with the therapist. The exercise, tasks, and language rehabilitation sessions were carried out concurrently every day, on a rotation basis.

My appetite was normal. I was always hungry, my body probably demanding nutrients to heal. During the hospitalization, I finished all my meals, but due to being diagnosed with hypertension during daily blood pressure measurements, my diet was changed to a low-salt one.

The only way to reduce salt was to cut the amount of miso soup in half and to change to a low-sodium type of bread. The flavor did not change at all, so I did not mind. I thought it was a healthy and tasty meal that would not worsen my condition. I enjoyed it like an in-flight meal on a plane. I was happy.

The one thing I had trouble with was using the toilet. I struggled with the first bowel movement I had after being hospitalized. Getting to the bathroom in a wheelchair was fine. However, not having any indication of anything coming, despite straining, was painful. Even after regaining the ability to walk a few days later, perhaps due to the poor mobility of the right side of my body, I struggled with the bowel movement.

I had never experienced such discomfort. It was so difficult and painful that I seriously thought I would have been better off if I hadn't survived (the stroke)! "I hate this!" I told the nurse and was given a laxative, which I immediately took. Little by little, small stools began to come out, and this problem too, slowly continued improving.

REHAB TRIALS AND MIRACLES

I was getting used to rehabilitation, and about five days had passed when I thought to myself 'I'm really doing the same thing every day'. That day, during the exercise part of rehabilitation, the physical therapist said, "Now, try moving your arm!'". I tried to lift my right arm and...managed a smooth motion."

Oh, my arm moved! I moved my arm!

I hadn't even tried hard, I just moved it lightly. It was just a small difference, but I could feel that my right arm moved. The previous day it had been so heavy that I could barely lift it, but now it moved naturally to just above my chest. It was only an additional 10 cm, but I was over the moon!

This was the moment a small ray of hope shone in my heart. I had found a light in the darkness. It was as if a door that had been tightly closed opened a little. My body is alive! The moment I realized this; I was convinced that I was going to be cured. I was on my way to recovery!

リハビリテーション実施計画書

患者ID	1576395	年齢	59	計画評価実施日：	2023年11月30日	急性期・外来等
氏名	黒米 髙広	性別	男			
主治医：		Ns:		OT:	ST:	MSW：	管理栄養士：

診断名・術式・障害名(発症日、手術日、診断日)	合併症・既往歴
主病名 脳梗塞 発症日：2023/11/26	なし

リスク管理：	安静度：血圧180以下、フリー
日常生活自立度：	B-2	認知症老人の日常生活自立度：	Ⅱa

評価項目・内容

- ☐ 意識障害(JCS) ☐ 1桁(軽度) ☐ 2桁(中等度) ☐ 3桁(重度)
- ☑ 認知機能　MMSE　25　/30点
- ☑ 高次脳機能障害
  - ☐ 記憶障害 ☐ 注意障害 ☐ 半側空間無視 ☐ 失行 ☐ 失認
  - ☐ 構成障害 ☐ 意思・意欲の障害 ☐ その他（　今後精査　）
- ☑ 言語障害
  - ☑ 構音障害 ☐ 運動性失語 ☐ 感覚性失語 ☐ 全失語 ☐ その他
- ☑ 中枢性麻痺(ステージ・グレード)
  - ☑ 右 ☐ 左　上肢：　Ⅵ　手指：　Ⅴ　下肢：　Ⅴ
- ☐ 感覚障害（☐ 表在覚 ☐ 深部覚　部位：　　　　　）
- ☐ 鈍麻（☐ 軽度 ☐ 中程度 ☐ 重度 ☐ 脱失 ☐ 過敏）しびれ

- ☐ 関節可動域制限　☐ 右 ☐ 左　部位：
- ☐ 筋柔軟性低下　部位：
- ☑ 筋力低下　部位：四肢、体幹
- ☑ 疼痛　程度、種類、部位：軽度頭痛
- ☐ 膨隆、浮腫　程度、部位：
- ☐ 荷重制限　☐ 免荷 ☐ 部分荷重(　　　　)
- ☐ 内部障害(☐心機能低下 ☐呼吸機能低下 ☐腎機能低下 ☐ その他)
- ☑ 耐久性低下　程度：中等度
- ☐ 摂食・嚥下障害：
- ☐ その他

		起居動作	☑ 自立 ☐ 部分介助 ☐ 全介助 ☐ 非実施	坐位保持	☑ 自立 ☐ 部分介助 ☐ 全介助 ☐ 非実施
基本動作		起立動作	☐ 自立 ☑ 部分介助 ☐ 全介助 ☐ 非実施	立位保持	☐ 自立 ☑ 部分介助 ☐ 全介助 ☐ 非実施
		屋内歩行	☐ 独立 ☑ 部分介助 ☐ 全介助 ☐ 非実施	（杖・装具：　　　　）	点滴棒

FIMの項目	現在の状態	本人・家族の希望
		本人：早く良くなりたい
食事	5 点	家族：未聴取
整容	1 点	
清拭	1 点	目標（1ヶ月）
更衣（上半身）	1 点	上肢機能向上
更衣（下半身）	1 点	病棟内日常生活の自立
トイレ動作	5 点	
排尿コントロール	6 点	
排便コントロール	6 点	
椅子移乗	5 点	目標（退院時）
トイレ移乗	5 点	応用動作の獲得
浴槽移乗	1 点	退院後の日常生活自立
移動	4 点	上記を目指し、状況に応じて1日20-40分のリハビリを1-2回程度行ないます。
階段	1 点	
運動項目 計 /91点	42 点	栄養
理解	6 点	身長： 172 cm 体重： 56 kg BMI： 18.929 kg/㎡
表出	6 点	標準体重：（ 65.1 ）kg ※身長測定が困難な場合は省略可
社会交流	5 点	栄養補給方法 ☐ 経口（☑ 食事、☐ 補助食品） ☐ 経管栄養
問題解決	5 点	☐ 静脈栄養（☐ 末梢、☐ 中心）
記憶	6 点	嚥下調整食の必要性：☑ 無 ☐ 有（学会分類コード　　　）
認知項目 計 /35点	28 点	栄養状態 ☑ 問題なし ☐ 低栄養 ☐ 低栄養リスク
総合計 /126点	70 点	☐ 過栄養　☐ その他（　　　）

本人・家族への説明日　2023年11月30日

本人・家族サイン　くろごめたかひろ　　説明者サイン

新規作成日：2021年03月29日
最終改訂日：2022年10月03日

The Power of Faith

After that day, I enjoyed my daily rehabilitation very much. It was not a sudden recovery, but I spent every day smiling. I felt relieved that I was on my way to recovery. I could trust in my body. The body is amazing. It is the miracle of life.

My body was really slowly recovering, everything little by little. The range of movement of my arms, the speed at which I could move them, and the work I could do with my hands, all came back little by little. Walking was also getting better and better. The weight of the right arm no longer bothered me. I felt comfortable with the rhythm of nature, and the speed of the changes.

I was deeply moved seeing myself gradually improving, smoothly and continuously. It felt like I'd been taught the true workings of my body, that I had never known before. The body becomes (more) mobile through use, doesn't it? Such wonder!

On the day I had the stroke, my body and tongue gradually stopped moving. I fell into the darkness of fear. But now, on the contrary, I am gradually starting to move again. A miraculous light shines, giving me strength, and I rise steadily, overflowing with smiles, as my body and tongue gradually begin to move again. It's a wonderful feeling. On this day, I asked ChatGPT to generate an image of the miracle of life.

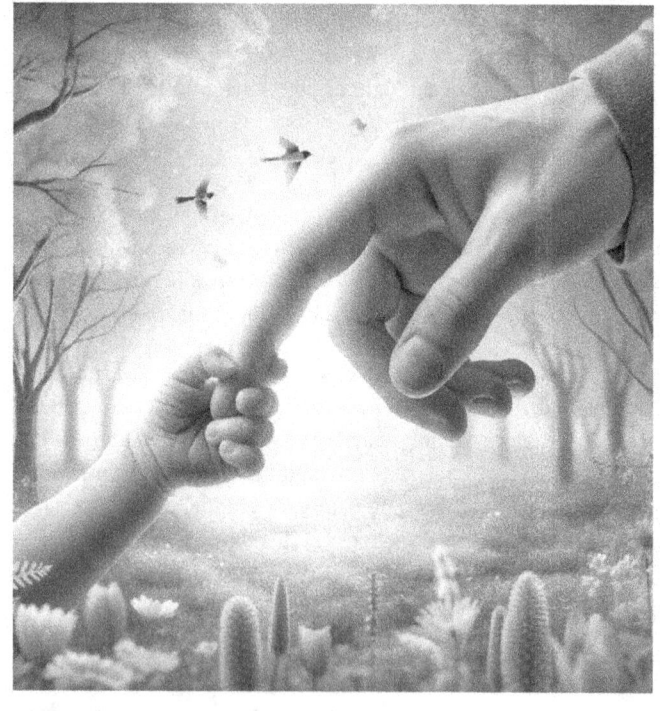

(ChatGPT generated image "Image of the Miracle of Life")

Rebirth

It is very fortunate that my memory and judgment were not affected. I remember being surprised by the changes in my body, and I can convey the trajectory of my recovery, which has been progressing smoothly.

I am lucky to be able to speak about the shock at the changes in my body, the sensations that stayed in my mind, and the smooth progression of my recovery.

It was only about three months, but it was wonderful to be able to enjoy rehabilitation and savor the changes in my body. Surely, babies must find moving their arms and legs enjoyable. I think I recovered thanks to the protection of my ancestors, especially my grandmother, Tome-san.

December 10, 2023 (Sun.) Discharge from the hospital

I was able to walk about a week after his hospitalization, and my rehabilitation progress was deemed to be satisfactory. After being discharged from the hospital, I would continue rehabilitation at home. The Christmas tree and Santa Claus at the hospital entrance saw me off as I headed home.

Even though I can walk, I still walk carefully because of my instability. I can't run or ride a bicycle. I still need practice writing characters, using chopsticks, and typing on the keyboard. For home rehabilitation, I take a walk every morning with a goal of reaching 8,000 steps. I also practice forming sounds, starting with hiragana and numbers, and later moving on to kanji (Chinese characters) every day.

When I visited the hospital for an outpatient rehabilitation visit half a month later, I had improved even further, so that visit was the only one I needed to have.

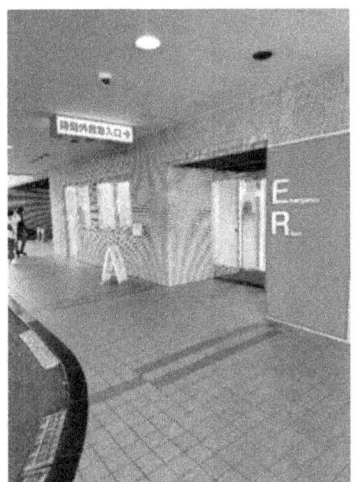

Entrance conveyed on November 26, 2023

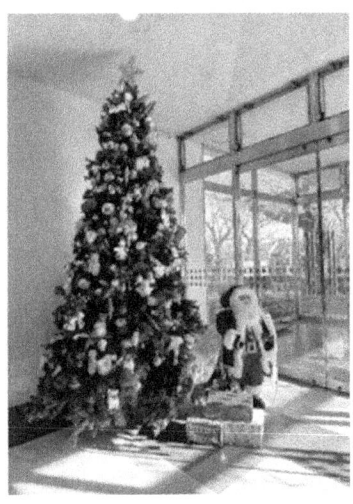

Hospital Entrance

The Power of Faith

Chapter 6
Learning to Type on the keyboard

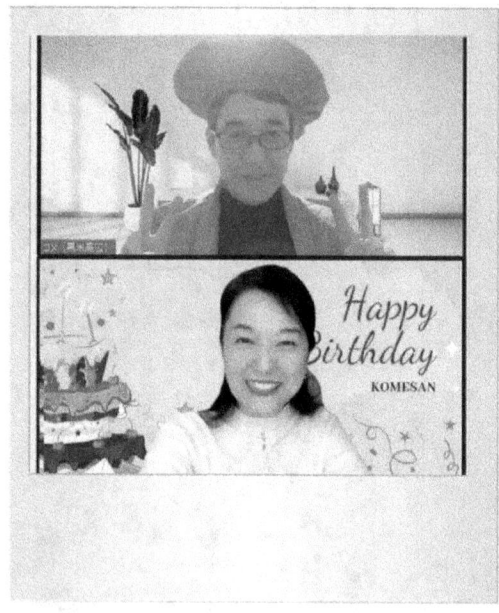

Chapter 6: Learning to Type on the Keyboard

The Joy of Being Able to Type on the Keyboard

My biggest problem was that I could no longer type on the keyboard.

I could manage to eat with a spoon and fork, but I had to type on the keyboard by hand. Even after a month of rehabilitation at home, I still cannot use a keyboard. My right arm gets tired, my fingers do not move well, and I catch other keys.

I continued to practice using the keyboard and writing. At a stationery store, I bought letter and number drills for young children and continued to write through them in pencil. In the beginning, I could not even write these simple letters and numbers well, which made me very sad. The only way forward, however, is to keep practicing. I persevered and gradually improved.

Miraculous Facebook Live

On January 30, 2024, the day I celebrated my 60th birthday, Ms. Tamaki Kuniyasu asked me to make a guest appearance on her Facebook Live. Ms. Kuniyasu had been worried about me after learning I had been hospitalized due to a stroke and asked me to join her. She recommended pine needle juice, which she herself drinks for her health.

I had no idea that I would be sharing about my stroke experience on Facebook Live, dressed in a red hat and red sleeveless kimono jacket. Thankfully, I discovered that I could type freely on the keyboard that day. I was completely cured within about three months of the onset of the disease. It's as if the right side of my body has been reborn.

Walking with Technology Again

I was deeply impressed by ChatGPT, a text-generating AI that debuted on November 30, 2022. Having studied electronics since middle school, learned about computers, and even built my own during my university days, I always believed that "a computer only outputs what you input." However, experiencing ChatGPT's responses made me realize how remarkable it is. I was amazed by the quality of the text and the speed of the answers. This, I thought, is what a truly advanced computer should be.

It can provide information, translate languages, assist with learning, generate and debug computer programs, engage in dialogue and counseling, offer creative ideas, do calculations and data analysis, offer strategies to improve SEO and websites, and even provide customer support. With the help of ChatGPT, I was able to start a seminar and finish then publish a Kindle manuscript in a short period of time.

The emergence of ChatGPT feels like glimpsing into the future of computers. Just as I was excited about computers and spent my middle school days learning about them, I'm excited about ChatGPT now. It allows anyone in the world to enjoy natural conversations with AI and learn from those conversations. "AI that converses with humans" will continue to evolve and have a lasting impact on the world.

I hope that Chat GPT will free people from tasks that they are not good at, so that they can concentrate on what they really want to do and truly enjoy the important moments in life.

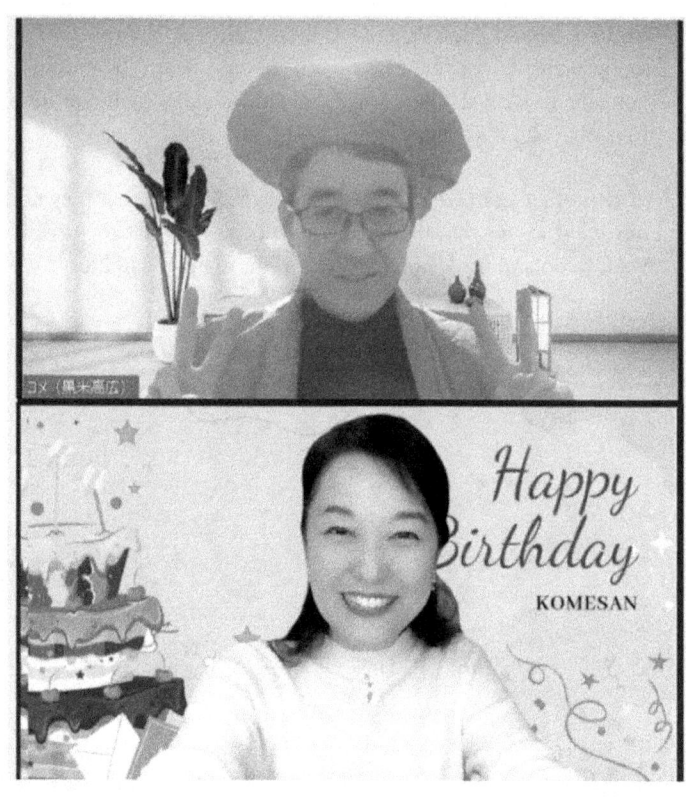

Screenshot of the Facebook Live of Tamaki Kuniyasu (below) the author (above)

The End of a Miracle, a New Beginning

When I experienced a sudden stroke, I fell into despair, and yet, how much it has brought me! I am grateful for the series of coincidences, the chain of miracles, and everything I have gained through this experience.

Below are some of the miracles and blessings I give thanks for:

- Realizing thanks to my routine that I can't write after waking up.
- Being able to call an ambulance for myself despite my speech becoming impaired.
- Receiving treatment for the stroke within 3 hours.
- Noticing small movements in my body during rehabilitation.
- Being able to trust in my body through these small movements.
- The faith that allowed me to keep going through rehabilitation.
- Being able to type on a keyboard again.
- Becoming a seminar lecturer in a short period using ChatGPT.
- Being able to publish on Kindle in a short period using ChatGPT.

No one knows when they will fall ill. I never thought I would have a stroke. If you notice any unusual movements or sensations in your body, please go to the hospital immediately. Don't just think, "I'll be fine." This is my message to you.

Afterword

Upon finishing this book, I am once more deeply aware of all the people who have supported me. It has been a miraculous thing to pull together. I would like to express my heartfelt gratitude to my family, friends, the staff at the holiday clinic, the emergency services, the hospital staff, the social networking community, and everyone else who was involved. I thank all the ancestors for the opportunity of our meeting.

Thank you to the doctor who saved my life with his proper judgment and prompt treatment. Thank you for the support from all the nurses, and physical, occupational, and speech therapists. It is because of all your support that I was able to make a full recovery. My heart overflows with gratitude.

The warm words I received from the SNS community not only made me smile but also gave me great encouragement to continue my recovery. Thank you very much.

My recovery went well and ChatGPT helped me a lot. Within a short period of time, I was able to prepare and conduct a seminar and write this book. I would like to thank all those who developed it; and hope that AI will encourage everyone to use their time wisely and experience a richer life.

Dear readers. I sincerely hope that this article will bring a little courage and hope to those who are concerned thinking that post-stroke symptoms cannot be cured, to those who are at risk of having a stroke, and to stroke patients as well as their families and loved ones. Thank you for reading through to the end. It would make me very happy if you could leave your thoughts and suggestions in the Amazon comments!

June 2024 Author

EXTERNAL LINKS

■Facebook
https://www.facebook.com/takahiro.kurogome

■X(旧twitter)
http://x.com/ktakahiro

■youtube
https://www.youtube.com/channel/UCYjybAJ88cmTeJ0j7UfvgVQ

■Instagram
https://www.instagram.com/kome_takahiro/

■Threads
https://www.threads.net/@kome_takahiro

■TikTok
https://www.tiktok.com/@kome339?_t=8mvzeNiVl7o&_r=1

■Clubhouse
https://www.joinclubhouse.com/@tar357

SPECIAL ACKNOWLEDGEMENTS

I would like to thank the many people who helped and enthusiastically supported me in the writing of this book. In particular, I would like to express our gratitude to Ms. Keiko Sato, the Kindle publishing producer. I am very grateful to her. I lost a family member to a subarachnoid hemorrhage, and she sympathized with my wish for many people to know about cerebral infarction, a type of stroke, and she took notes during our fun Zoom chats, even when I was engrossed in the conversation, so I could write the manuscript, which turned out better than I had imagined. Thank you very much. I am infinitely grateful for the opportunity to work with you.

Ms. Hiroko Iwasaki, representative of the General Association of Attractive Parenting Moms. Ms. Chie Satake, proprietress of the yakitori restaurant "Nihonbashi Torikei," e-book publication conceptor and writer, and certified instructor of the Attractive Parenting Association. She looked over the manuscript and gave us accurate and valuable advice. We are grateful to both for changing the structure and making it easier to read. Thank you for your support for this book. I would like to thank you from the bottom of my heart. Keiko Sato is also responsible for their Kindle publication. We are indebted to Ms. Keiko Iwasaki for the simultaneous publication of the English and Spanish versions. Thank you very much.

I would like to thank Katsunari Tanaka, founder of Clubhouse "GIFLabO", communications marketer and creator of the card game "GIFT", and all the moderators. I laughed every morning in my boring hospital bed. I am very happy to have met "Noripi & Dora-chan". They were incredibly funny. I loved it! Thank you very much.

Yumi Tanabe says, "I'm just an ordinary housewife who gets up a little early. The reason she moved my schedule up a day for the "Beebe Fuku no Kami Work" was because she heard my grandmother Tome's voice saying, "Hurry up and do it! I laughed in agreement. I think it was my grandmother Tome-san (494) who worried about me all the time after my parents divorced and saved me from a stroke. Yumi-san told me in her blessing work that I (246) have the item 4 (talkative), which has been a great encouragement to me in writing this book. My strong supporter is Tome-san. Thank you for the opportunity to meet you. I was also able to meet Yumi-san in real life at the "Nagi Matsuri" (2024/5/21-24) hosted by Yumi-san. I have good memories of "5/23 night of Adult Serious Play". Thank you very much.

stroke at noon on 5/23. At the evening's adult serious play, we spent the night alone in the same room with Mr. Nagi, sharing a futon side by side. The next morning, 5/24, we sat down on the landing of a boat on the Montiches beach, which stretched out in front of our accommodations, and talked alone with each other while looking out at the sea. The morning sea breeze blew pleasantly through the intersection of each other's single lives. It is a deep and intense time that we can understand each other because we are of the same age. We look forward to seeing more of our combined futures. This occasion was wonderfully refreshing and allowed me to write my Kindle manuscript, feeling good. Thank you very much.

Noripi (Noriko Narita) is a GIFLab moderator who supports overseas entrepreneurship, trades medical equipment, manages a real estate company, and conducts organizational analysis (personality psychology). We were able to meet again in real life at noon on May 23, also at the "Nagi Festival. We spent the rest of the evening having a real night out and chatting, and the next morning, 5/24, Noripi was live chatting on the open LINE from her hammock. It was interesting to hear him right next to us. After lunch, we went with him to Meitokuji Temple in Innoshima (Onomichi City), which is open once every 33 years. I was thrilled with the long drive. It is a wonderful memory. It was with a sense of excitement and thrill that I was able to write this book. Thank you very much.

Akari Taniyama, a friend of GIFLabo fan and representative of Anela, who "lights the light of hope in your heart" with her healing pastel art & mental meditation mandala art. She called me the day I was hospitalized, worried about me. It made me very happy! The feedback and frank impressions you shared about the first draft of this book were incredibly valuable. Thank you very much.

Masamichan (Mr. Takumi Nakagawa), whose hobby is LINE consulting, is a GIFLab moderator, and I am grateful for his help on LINE. We met for the first time at the graduation ceremony and were also together at the event the next day. A week later, he was the first to comment on my Facebook post that I had been hospitalized due to a stroke, which made me very happy. Thank you so much.

Ms. Tamaki Kuniyasu is a vocalist and happy voice trainer. She lost her father to a stroke. She was very concerned about my health after the stroke and taught me how to make pine needle juice. I was very happy! Tamaki invited me as a guest to her Facebook Live and sang Happy Birthday to me. I am happy. Thank you to everyone who warmly watched me at the live performance. Thank you very much. I am glad to be alive.

Toshihiko (Toshi) Kano, AIxWeb3 era and AI practitioner, and Shuichi (Shu-chan) Kido, reverse entrepreneurship producer, who taught us the basics of ChatGPT and business ideas. I learned a lot and became a ChatGPT seminar instructor. Thank you very much.

And for drafting chapters and sentences, pointing out and correcting mistakes. Thanks to ChatGPT for their tremendous contribution; without ChatGPT, I could not have completed this book in a short time.

HIRO (Hiroshi Saito) of AI Support AI HEROES, for looking over my 40,000-word Kindle manuscript and immediately sending me his feedback and valuable suggestions. Thank you very much.

My ancestors Toru Kobayashi (paternal grandfather), Sen Kobayashi (paternal grandmother), Kanichiro Ishiwatari (maternal grandfather), Tome Ishiwatari (maternal grandmother), and my father Eisaku Kobayashi whom I could not meet again before his death. I am truly blessed. I would like to thank all our ancestors for connecting us.

AUTHOR'S PROFILE

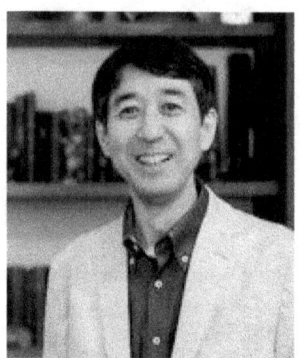

Takahiro Kurogome

Born in Tokyo in January 1964. Lives and works in Tokyo. Became interested in electronics and computers when he was in the second grade of junior high school and studied electronics for six months through correspondence courses. He went on to a technical high school and technical college to realize his dream of becoming an electrical engineer. Developed an automatic testing device while working for a company and was shocked by ChatGPT. Hospitalized for 2 weeks due to a stroke in November 2023. In February 2024, he started ChatGPT seminars upon his retirement. His nickname is Kome. He loves coffee. His hobby is listening to Mozart. He has written two books. The 44 Books I Read in the New Corona Disaster - I Started a Rich Life by Reading + Taking Action" (2021, kindle) and" The Power to Believe - You Can Be a Miracle Worker, Too! ～(2024, kindle).

The Power of Faith

Harness the Power to Create Miracles!

(2024, kindle)

Publication date June 23, 2024,

Japanese edition, first published

Author Takahiro Kurogome

All rights to this e-book are reserved by the author. Reproduction, alteration, reprinting, duplication, distribution, transmission, or reprinting on a website, in whole or in part, of this book is prohibited. With exceptions, this is prohibited by copyright law. Please contact us via Facebook Messenger.

Copyright © 2024 Takahiro Kurogome All rights reserved.